DISCLAIMER

This book is not intended as a substitute for the medical advice of physicians. You should regularly consult a physician in matters relating to your health, particularly with respect to any symptoms that may require diagnosis or medical attention. Let your physician know if you plan to make changes to your lifestyle or diet. Never stop taking a prescribed medicine without consulting your physician.

Read the research and other sources used to prepare this guide (most with live links). Visit the page for **supplemental info** at http://www.cheatsheetstore.com

It's all free!

First get just an inkling how complex your body is
Learn what inflammation is
Understand the things that cause chronic inflammation
See how chronic inflammation damages your body
Learn the things you can do to improve your health
You cannot effectively treat your chronic disease until you treat your chronic inflammation.

Get Yourself Well

No matter what health problem you might have, there is one condition which you have the power to manage which can improve your health. The condition you must manage is chronic inflammation. Yes you have it. It is almost impossible in this modern world to be free of chronic inflammation. If you have no signs or symptoms of any kind, you just don't have them yet. You will understand this as you learn about what causes chronic inflammation.

If you have a chronic ailment which just won't improve, you may find that managing your chronic inflammation is just what you need. Chronic inflammation is making your condition worse. It may even be causing your condition. Decreasing chronic inflammation is a powerful way to improve your health because it helps your body operate as it should. Then your body can make itself better.

Controlling chronic inflammation can give meaning to the old saying, "add years to your life and life to your years."

The list of diseases that chronic inflammation affects - either causes or makes worse - is long and frightening. Here are a few.

cancer	liver disease
heart disease	psoriasis
diabetes	migraines
Alzheimer's	periodontal disease
asthma	lupus
stroke	irritable bowel syndrome
arthritis	Crohn's disease
kidney disease	PCOS (polycystic ovary
osteoporosis	syndrome)
hypertension	Parkinson's
Multiple sclerosis	depression
gout	lung disease (like COPD)

Inflammation is an immune response of the body. It is meant to protect the body and help it heal. We've all experienced some form of inflammation.

Sprain your ankle and it hurts and swells

Scrape your knee and it gets red and swells

Wake up with a sore throat

These are all examples of inflammation that is normal and healthy. Inflammation is the beginning of the healing process. This was

2

recognized by Hippocrates long ago, around 400 B.C.

The body system that controls inflammation is the immune system. The basic parts of the immune system are:

- lymphatic system - lymph nodes and vessels which carry lymph fluid around the body
- spleen - filters the blood for foreign matter
- tonsils and thymus - make white blood cells (leukocytes) and antibodies
- bone marrow - makes blood cells
- white blood cells - kill foreign organisms

The usual signs of inflammation are pain and tenderness, redness, heat, and edema (swelling). Inflammation is often unpleasant but it is necessary.

There are three usual causes of inflammation.

1. Foreign organisms or pathogens. The three most common types are bacteria, viruses and fungi. Someone coughs, you breathe in the germs, inflammation begins. You eat food that has started to spoil and the bacteria inflames your intestines.

2. Injury. You break a bone. You get a splinter in your finger.

3. Irritation. Foreign matter gets into your body or comes in contact with your body. You are near a campfire and breathe in the smoke. You have a sensitivity to tomatoes and accidentally eat some in a salad.   You touch poison ivy. Irritation can be seen as an injury on a small scale because an irritant is damaging cells. Like sand irritating an oyster and causes a pearl to form. When your cells are irritated they don't make pearls, they make inflammation.

Here is an overview of how inflammation works.

A pathogen or irritant enters the body or you are injured and inflammatory chemicals are released into your blood. Those chemicals activate other chemicals and specialized cells. Each of those cells and chemicals, in turn, activate other cells and chemicals. It is a little like a snowball rolling downhill, picking up momentum and bulk. This process is often referred to as the inflammation cascade.

Each chemical and type of cell has a purpose related to solving the problem. Everything does it's specialized job, which broadly will fall into one of three categories:

- Kill pathogens
- Clean up dead organic matter
- Bring nutrients and raw materials to the area to begin healing

Once the problem is dealt with, the cascade reverses itself. The inflammatory chemicals subside and anti-inflammatory chemicals are released and begin to shut down the process.

This is called acute inflammation because it is usually short term. It deals with a single problem and goes away when the problem does. It's a good thing. Inflammation goes bad when it doesn't go away or when it starts up again constantly. It can cause a lot of damage to your body and even become less effective at doing it's own job.

The good news is that it has been shown that reducing chronic inflammation can improve, avoid or even eliminate many conditions.

Basic Chemistry of Inflammation

When inflammation is required the cascade begins and cells at the site begin production or increase of cytokines like il-1 and il-8, mast cells, basophils and platelets.

Cytokines provide communication between cells and include interleukins, interferons and growth factors. Some switch cells on or off to begin or stop their function. Other cytokines attract other chemicals or different types of leukocytes. Interleukin is usually abbreviated with IL and the number that identifies that specific chemical like the il-1 and il-8 mentioned above.

Many of these early responders initiate the release of histamine.

Histamine is a chemical made and released by mast cells and basophils. When released histamine dilates blood vessels and increases the permeability of nearby cells. In the blood vessel wall this means fluid can seep out into the surrounding tissue. This is a cause of puffiness in an allergy. Histamine also stimulates release of more cytokines.

Mast cells are found throughout the body in tissues and in the blood. When they are activated they may cause an immediate allergic response or they may begin synthesis of cytokines and chemokines. Some specifie functions they contribute to are building immunity, fighting parasites, tissue repair, angiogenesis, and they help regulate the immune system.

Platelets   are very small cells whose main function is to stop bleeding. They also attract leukocytes and other platelets to an injury or inflammation. They may release pro-inflammatory, anti-inflammatory and angiogenic chemicals based upon the environment.

Leukocytes are white blood cells. They are important in the inflammation cascade and the different types of leukocytes perform different functions.

Basophils are a type of leukocyte which eat some types of bacteria, foreign material <u>and other cells</u>.

Eosinophils are not very numerous (normally less than 4% of total leukocytes). They kill some bacteria, destroy some foreign material and are especially useful against parasites.

Monocytes are white blood cells that circulate in the blood, but enter tissues at problem sites and become macrophages.

Neutrophils are the most common type of leukocyte. When you have an injury or infection they divide to increase their numbers and eat foreign matter.

The leukocytes known as lymphocytes come in 2 types: B and T. B types produce antibodies. The T cells are able to recognize surface proteins on other cells and when they run into something that shouldn't be there, a lymphocyte releases chemicals which kill it on contact or helps kill it.

Antibodies are specialized proteins which the body uses to identify and destroy foreign matter, which may include non-organic things (dust in your eye or dirt in a wound) or organic matter (bacteria, viruses, fungi, dead cells). There is an indefinite number of types of antibody as they are created in response to each new foreign material that enters the body.

Phagocyte describes a type of cell function. Phagocytes ingest foreign material and cell debris. Different types of white blood cells can act as phagocytes: neutrophils, eosinophils and monocytes.

On the heels of the initial chemicals, others are released as the cascade gains momentum.

Macrophages are cells that clean up debris (dead cells) and pathogens (bacteria,etc). The process is called phagocytosis. They basically envelop the pathogen or debris and dissolve it using enzymes and peroxides.

A macrophage can destroy up to 100 bacteria (or other items) <u>before dying from it's own</u>

<u>digestive juices</u>. Obviously, it brews up some pretty potent stuff. Some macrophages are fixed in one location while others travel throughout the blood stream looking for problems.

The above is the best known of the duties of the macrophage. However, recent research shows macrophages can be activated or turned on by different chemicals. When turned on by either il-4 or glucocorticoids a macrophage does not do a good job of destroying invaders but produces compounds that are involved in creating an extracellular matrix used in tissue repair.

TNF alpha stands for tumor necrosis factor alpha. It is a cytokine that, among other things, signals where all the other chemicals that respond to injury should go - it identifies the site where inflammation is needed.

CRP is c-reactive protein. It is made in the liver in response to levels of il-6. It attaches to cells and some bacteria. It marks things for the macrophages to destroy. There is a low level of CRP in the blood at all times. In the presence of infection or injury the level of CRP can increase 1000 fold in 48 hours or less.

Interleukin-6 is a cytokine that influences monocytes to an area of injury where they become macrophages and it also triggers production of CRP.

Chemokines are cytokines that specialize in chemotaxis, which is to chemically alter the environment to attract or repel cells.

Bradykinines are chemicals that dilate blood vessels and increases their permeability.

These are not the only chemicals that come to play but some of the most important that are known. These are not the only things they do, either. The cells and chemicals in our body are all masters at multi-tasking. You should have an idea now how complicated the body and inflammation are and how it is possible for something in one part of the body to have influence over what happens in another seemingly unrelated part of the body. And these chemical changes all lead to many physical changes.

Some Physical Changes Caused by These Chemicals

ROS, reactive oxygen species, are better known as free radicals. These are chemicals created when cells turn oxygen into water (to produce energy). ROS are waste or left overs from this process. Other sources of ROS include radiation like UV light, toxic chemicals and drugs.

Formation of ROS increases oxygen consumption, oxidation of glucose, and creation of superoxides which are chemically altered into still other chemicals. Some of these chemicals dissolve pathogens and debris and are not a problem in correct quantities for the situation.

Malondialdehyde (MDA) is a by-product of ROS interacting with polyunsaturated fats in your body. The MDA can evolve to many other things. When it interacts with your DNA it creates at least one compound that is mutagenic which means it can cause mutations to your DNA. As a mutagen, it also has potential to be carcinogenic (cause cancer).

There is vasodilation in inflammation. The blood vessels in the inflamed area get larger, usually referring to the very small vessels at the site. This causes a greater blood flow to the area of inflammation, resulting in redness and heat. This dilation is in part triggered by histamines, prostaglandins, nitric oxide and bradykinines.

There is vascular stasis: the flow of blood slows down in the area of inflammation to make it easier for leukocytes to leave the blood vessel and go into the injured or threatened tissue.

Chemicals (again including histamines and bradykinines, plus leukotrienes and cytokines like il-1 and TNF and more), cause the endothelial cells on the walls of the blood vessels to contract, which causes them to become "leaky". This is called vascular permeability. Fluids and cells can pass through the vessel wall which is something they can't normally do.

How Does All This Harm Your Body?

An inflammation cascade requires energy to begin and end. It is work. Just like driving a car 100,000 miles will cause more wear than driving 10,000 miles. As the saying goes, it's not the years it's the miles. That's just the beginning of the damage.

Phagocytes destroy or dispose of debris but they also destroy adjacent cells. With the occasional acute inflammation it can be considered acceptable collateral damage. When it is chronic it adds to the burden on the body to recuperate.

ROS (the free radicals) act upon molecules of lipids, proteins, carbohydrates and nucleic acids. The ROS are like little zombies. When they bump into another molecule they take a bite and steal a hydrogen atom. That destabilizes the other molecule and it becomes a free radical. A chain reaction results. The body has natural scavengers of the ROS but if ROS production gets too prolific it can cause an imbalance. This is called oxidative stress.

As noted, the c-reactive protein is always in the blood at a low level but can jump a whopping 1000 fold in a couple of days! It has also been demonstrated that high levels of CRP are a good predictor of heart and other cardiovascular problems. Yet it is not the super high levels that is a good predictor. It is a day to day level that is above what is normal which indicates cardiac problems in your future and that is what you have when you have chronic inflammation. The mystery is this: is CRP a cause or effect? No one knows whether CRP rise is because of inflammation or if it causes inflammation. It could be both. For our practical purposes it doesn't matter. We don't want either.

The strong chemicals that are produced to dissolve debris can cause ulceration of local tissues. Ulceration is an injury and begins another cascade.

Cellular damage sometimes leads to vascular insufficiency which means the local blood supply is not adequate. Inadequate amounts of blood and oxygen reach the area and this can cause damage and cell death and a new cascade begins.

Angiogenesis is the creation of new blood vessels including entire networks of vessels. This is useful when blood flow has been compromised as it often is with inflammation, but when it happens too often it may cause problems. Angiogenesis happens to be a standard occurrence in cancer to feed the runaway cells. One theory says angiogenesis either causes or speeds up Alzheimer's. Angiogenesis is also a key component of diabetic retinopathy and arthritis. Angiogenesis seems to be one of those things that is great when needed but if it shows up without a need, it tends to be bad news. Inflammation encourages it.

Fibrosis or scarring occurs when injuries don't heal exactly right and repeated injury (inflammation) in the same location can cause fibrosis. Within the tissues, fibrosis becomes a new source of irritation and inflammation.

Resistance means that something doesn't respond to a cue the way it should. For example someone with recurring headaches may take care of it with one aspirin at first. Months later it may take 2 aspirins. Months after that it may take 3.

Insulin resistance seems to be getting more common and is seriously bad news. Insulin resistance is closely associated with chronic inflammation. Here is a simple explanation of how insulin resistance occurs.

Sugar is to your body what gasoline is to your car. It is the fuel that keeps us going. Some of everything you eat turns to sugar and goes into your blood stream and the blood carries the sugar fuel to all the cells of the body.

Insulin is made in the pancreas and it's big purpose is to attach to sugar in the blood and help it get into all your cells where it can be used. Sugar can't get into the cell without insulin.

Each cell has a set capacity for sugar. It can only hold a certain amount at one time. Just like a quart jar will hold a quart and not a drop more.

If there is still sugar in the blood it works a little like a thermostat to signal the pancreas to pump more insulin so the sugar can get into the cells. But the sugar won't go into a cell if the cell is at capacity so the pancreas will pump still more insulin.

Eventually resistance develops. More insulin is needed to get sugar into cells even when the cells have available space.

Over time insulin production will begin to decrease and the cells will not get the energy they need to function properly. This keeps organs and the body in general from working properly. Eventually the pancreas will stop producing insulin completely. When it gets to that point, you have diabetes.

Research has shown that several chemicals released during inflammation suppress cell response to insulin. Inflammation is intended to be temporary, after all. So the likelihood for insulin resistance increases as chronic inflammation increases.

On the other hand, insulin resistance can cause inflammation. A key inflammatory cytokine, interleukin-1-beta is switched on by a protein FOX01. Insulin resistance increases the activity of FOX01.

So once they begin, chronic inflammation and insulin resistance sustain one another.

High blood sugar does even more damage. It seems high blood sugar is not compatible with nitric oxide. When blood sugar goes up, nitric oxide decreases. That is important because nitric oxide allows blood vessels to flex and dilate. When there isn't enough it causes high blood pressure which can injure organs all over your body.

We are not finished with sugar. But first, good news. Don't worry so much about cholesterol, any of it. You probably are aware that there are two general types of cholesterol, HDL, high density lipid, and LDL, low density lipid. Once upon a time it was thought all cholesterol was bad. That would actually be strange because 75% of the cholesterol in your body is made by your body. Later it was decided that LDL is bad and HDL is good. That has been even more refined. LDL comes in different sizes. Large molecule LDL is good for you. It is small dense LDL molecules that are associated with health issues. This is related to sugar because high blood sugar raises levels of small dense molecule LDL. We don't know why, yet, but they go together – high blood sugar and high levels of small dense LDL. To put them together just a bit more, as the excess sugar is coursing through your vessels it is inflaming the walls of your vessels with what are essentially scratches. The small LDL gets lodged into these grooves and begins a buildup that ends in a heart attack or stroke.

When sugar cannot get into the cells and your body decides to give up trying another problem shows up. Excess sugar does not get excreted. It is stored in fat cells.

Fat cells, adipocytes, store excess energy that won't fit into the cells, as fat. Fat is stored in the form of fatty acids called triglycerides. Adipose tissue, or a group of fat cells, is found between the skin and muscle (subcutaneous fat) and around the organs in the main body cavities (visceral fat, primarily in the abdominal cavity).

Visceral fat has been linked to increased risk for cardiovascular disease and type 2 diabetes and to metabolic disturbances. In women, it is also associated with breast cancer and the need for gallbladder surgery.

Cortisol resistance is yet another problem. Cortisol is a steroid hormone produced in the adrenal glands. It's production is influenced by

fasting or eating
exercise
stress
just waking up (when it is normally highest).

Cortisol helps store and move fat and matures young fat cells. It can suppress the immune system and increase appetite. Excess cortisol also breaks down collagen which is needed for healthy skin, so it not only does hidden damage but makes you look older.

As more fat (unused sugar) accumulates in the body, cortisol begins to store it in the abdomen (visceral fat). Cortisol is made from cortisone by action of an enzyme made by fat cells. Visceral fat cells produce more of this enzyme than the fat under your skin. Also, there are 4 times more cortisol receptors in visceral fat cells which may increase it's fat accumulating effect.

So cortisol encourages and sustains it's own

over-production by storing more visceral fat.

The greatest initiator of cortisol production is stress. Stress increases cortisol levels and long term high levels of stress can result in cortisol resistance which increases cortisol production which will contribute to chronic inflammation and insulin resistance.

Cortisol production is not the only way fat cells contribute to chronic inflammation. In the past, it was thought that fat cells were for storing fat and nothing more. Recent research has shown that is not true.

Adipocytes — especially abdominal fat cells — are active and act as an endocrine organ, producing hormones and other substances that affect our health. So visceral fat disrupts normal hormone balance and functioning and the more visceral fat there is, the more disruption there is. Visceral fat also pumps out the inflammatory cytokines TNF and il-6.

Fat cells can actually be so over-filled with fatty acids that they burst. Excess fat cells can also swell and shut off local blood supply to small vessels. That keeps blood and oxygen from getting the those cells and they die. Cell death from poor circulation and burst cells both begin new cascades of inflammation.

Besides fat cells and stress increasing cortisol production, so does lack of sleep. More excess cortisol equals more damage. At the same time, lack of adequate sleep decreases production of the growth hormone which in adults is needed to thicken skin, strengthen bones and increase muscle mass.

Lack of sleep puts more stress on the body and whether due to inflammation or something else, studies show that people who don't sleep enough are more likely to develop all types of disease and live shorter lives. Your body does routine tissue repairs during sleep. It can't happen if you don't get enough sleep.

Compare it to having a flat tire. Instead of repairing it you inflate it just enough to drive a block and it goes flat again and you inflate enough to go another block. Eventually, driving with too little air will damage the tire beyond usability. If you repaired the tire and inflated it properly it would last much longer.

Recall that inflammation is a natural function of the immune system. So it is important that 70% or more of the immune system is within the digestive system (as lymph tissue and white cells). Of course the digestive system is also a major route for inflammatory substances to get into your body. When there is trouble in your digestive system it should come as no surprise that it can throw your immune system out of whack and lead to many other problems including chronic inflammation.

There is a condition known as leaky gut which describes an unhealthy digestive system which allows matter from the digestive system to leak back into the tissues and blood stream. This matter will include pathogens and debris, both of which will cause more inflammatory cascades which is another instance of the problem sustaining itself.

The liver is vital and can both contribute to, and suffer from, chronic inflammation. The liver has over 500 functions including

Assimilates and stores fat-soluble vitamins
Creates bile needed for digestion
Filters blood
Metabolizes fats, proteins, and carbohydrates
Metabolizes hormones and foreign chemicals
Metabolizes internally-produced wastes,
Produces urea (a primary waste product, flushed from the body in urine)
Purifies and clears waste products, and toxins
Regulates and secretes substances important to maintain body functions and health

Stores important nutrients such as glycogen, glucose, vitamins, and minerals
Synthesizes blood proteins including CRP

———

With so many vital functions, it is extremely important that the liver work properly. When the liver is unable to do what it is intended to do it can affect every other part of your body.

One potential liver problem is related to fat storage. The liver stores fat cells. When there are too many fat cells, the liver stores too many and it can lead to a diseased liver that doesn't work properly. It's a medical condition known simply as fatty liver disease and anything with ability to cause your liver to fail is potentially deadly.

Inflammation creates a lot of debris and toxins which need to go through the liver. Excess amounts of waste such as that produced by continuous inflammation can over work the liver. If the liver doesn't do a good job of eliminating waste it makes another burden of foreign toxin being re-circulated and the immune system must deal with it by it's usual method, inflammation.

How Diet Contributes to Inflammation

Your diet has a lot of influence on chronic inflammation. Inflammation begins with chemicals. Chemicals in your body are derived from what you put in your body - foods, liquids and the nutrients within them. Some foods are inflammatory, while other foods are anti-inflammatory. So what you eat can directly help or hurt.

A part of everything you eat is converted to sugar and goes into your blood. Sugar is what the body uses for energy. Sugar becomes a problem when you get too much sugar too fast. You've read what happens when there is too much sugar too fast.

One of the most potentially damaging "foods" you can eat is pure sugar. The closer a substance is, mechanically and chemically, to glucose (blood sugar), the faster it gets into the blood. Sugar goes directly into the blood, gives you a fast blood sugar high and can make it difficult for the body (pancreas) to keep up. Whenever you add sugar to coffee, tea, cereal or anything you increase the potential for becoming insulin resistant and eventually diabetic. The same goes for slightly altered sugar, like doughnut icing.

The white sugar most of us eat has another problem. It is processed. Processed food has been altered. It is less complex chemically than raw food. Less complex means easier to digest, faster to digest, faster to convert into blood sugar.

Simple carbohydrates (processed foods) are everywhere. The average diet in the United States is filled with simple carbs, with many coming from grains and their products. This includes wheat (flour, bread, pasta), rice, and corn. Pretty much all snack foods, cereals and baked goods use processed ingredients and convert to blood sugar quickly. Most condiments are processed. These can all give you a high blood sugar.

Along with excess sugar, transfats are the next villain to consider. They are not always announced as transfats, however. Look for hydrogenated or partially hydrogenated oils - same thing. Don't assume there is no transfat if a package says transfat free. Make sure it is not on the list of ingredients. "Transfat Free" can legally be placed on a package if the food contains less than 0.5 grams of transfat per serving. A serving can be whatever the manufacturer decides. A newer related substance is interesterified fats.

Transfats increase LDL the "bad" cholesterol LDL. They make some of the LDL worse - make it into smaller denser particles that are more likely to cause plaque build up in your arteries. Transfats increase triglycerides in your blood which contributes to atherosclerosis. Transfats also damage the cell lining of blood vessels and that causes inflammation.

Another big problem with most diets is corn. Corn is not bad in and of itself. It's more the by products of corn that create the problem. Corn is very high in omega-6 fatty acid.

You need omega-6. You also need omega-3. Both are essential fatty acids which means your body does not make them so you need to consume them. Your system is designed to work with a specific balance or ratio of the two. Studies show that positive health results can be obtained by a diet where the ratio of omega-6 : omega-3 is within the range of 1:1 to 5:1. Estimates for the average diet in the United States place the ratio of the average diet in the range of 15:1 to 16.7:1. Some person's diets have a ratio of 30:1. The simple explanation of why this is unhealthy is the fact that omega-6 is inflammatory; omega-3 is anti-inflammatory.

Corn is everywhere. It is cheap, so corn starch, corn oil and corn syrup are used in most processed foods. In spite of the fact that corn is a grain, not a vegetable, very often when you see an ingredient listed as vegetable oil, it is corn oil or contains corn oil. So a standard diet loads your system with omega-6 many times per day and seldom adds omega-3.

Sensitivity to a food is another potential diet related problem. Essentially a sensitivity is a very mild allergy. The sensitivity may be so subtle that you don't notice it as it fuels chronic inflammation each time you eat the offending food.

It may come as a surprise but potatoes are potentially very dangerous. There have been no reported severe cases (multiple illness and death) for many years but it used to happen. If you have a potato with green under the skin or beginning to sprout, cut off that part. It is where the potato is beginning to grow that makes the toxin as a defense against insects.

Simply as an example of sensitivity consider the potato and it's family. The potato is a member of a family of plants that produce a toxin. They are the solanaceae plants, the nightshade family. Other plants in this family are peppers, eggplant, tomatoes and tobacco.

Don't just stop eating these plants. It is esti-mated that only between 1-3% of the popula-tion is sensitive to plants in the nightshade family. If you have no sensitivity to them, no problem. Among other things, tomatoes are high in lutein and peppers are high in vita-min C.   So they are good to eat if you're not sensitive.

Slight sensitivity is probably more prevalent than most people realize.   Some of the more common sensitivities and allergies are to wheat, dairy, shell fish and peanuts.

If a person with an allergy to a food eats that food, they can die. A person with a severe allergy can die from kissing someone who has eaten the food they are allergic to.   If you have a severe allergy to a food you probably know it. If you have a sensitivity it may be so subtle you seldom notice any effect.

Even if you only have sensitivity every time you eat the offending food you are fueling inflammation. If you have a problem of any kind when you eat a specific food, or you catch yourself saying "It doesn't agree with me," you may be sensitive.   The problem may be rash, itch, abdominal discomfort, headache, drowsiness, gas or can't sleep. Basically, anything that isn't normal.

Alcohol isn't exactly a food but it enters your body the same way and it definitely deserves a mention. There is no doubt that long term alcohol use can result in severe liver damage and digestive system ulcers.

Recently another health issue was brought to light. It was shown that a single binge could cause leaky gut (mentioned earlier) and put pathogens from the gut into the blood stream which will cause an inflammation cascade. Since pathogens are getting into the blood it may lead to dangerous sensitivities later because the immune system will manufacture antibodies. It seems likely that continued use below binge levels can also cause leaky gut related problems.

Alcohol is the primary cause of pancreatitis (which interferes with insulin production). It can cause the stomach to over produce stomach acid and lead to irritation. Alcohol can inflame the liver and cause it to store fat. It can cause blood pressure to rise.

Smoking is an incredibly important source of chronic inflammation. It damages your lungs' natural cleaning and repair system and traps cancer-causing chemicals in your lungs.

Cilia are tiny hairs which line the upper airways and protect against infection.

A healthy respiratory system has a thin layer of mucous and thousands of these cilia lining the insides of your breathing passages. The mucous traps dirt and pollution you breathe in, and the cilia move together like a wave to push the debris-filled mucous out of your lungs. You cough, then swallow or spit up the mucous, and the dirt is out of your lungs. Smoking destroys the cilia.

With your respiratory cleaning and repair system damaged, germs, dirt and chemicals from cigarette smoke stay inside your lungs. Cigarette smoke contains over 4,800 chemicals — 69 are known to cause cancer. Smoking is directly responsible for approximately 90 percent of lung cancer deaths and 80-90 percent of COPD (emphysema and chronic bronchitis) deaths.

Alveoli are small air sacs in the lungs where oxygen enters the blood. Smoke causes the alveoli to harden. That's an injury and causes inflammation. Every particle of debris that stays in the lungs and every molecule of toxic chemical inhaled is an irritant and begins a new cascade of inflammation.

Another contributor to chronic inflammation is stress. This includes both physical stress like an athlete might have from extreme work-outs and mental stress like anyone might get from money or relationship worries. It has long been accepted that stress is unhealthy and recently research discovered at least one way it probably contributes to poor health when you are 'sick'.

Whether stress is physical or mental, it triggers what is known as the fight or flight response and a natural result of this is the release of adrenalin into the body. When you have any infection part of the inflammatory response is to release il-6 into the blood. Recall that il-6 is an inflammatory chemical and helps begin inflammatory cascades. It has been shown that increased adrenalin in the blood, which occurs when a person has an infection, will increase the production of il-6 by 40 times.

Here is a quick recap of major points:

Chronic inflammation results from chemicals creating, depleting or otherwise acting on cells and other chemicals.

The chemical reactions of inflammation are triggered by injury, pathogens and irritation to any degree anywhere in the body.

Chemicals involved with inflammation must work together. Too much or too little of one chemical can change everything.

Inflammation creates free radicals and they are normal, but excess free radicals from chronic inflammation cause damage that leads to more inflammation and oxidative stress.

Fat cells encourage inflammation in multiple ways and visceral fat cells are the worst.

Chronic inflammation promotes resistance to insulin and cortisol and those resistances promote chronic inflammation.

When one system in the body doesn't work right, it puts a work overload on other systems and eventually can cause other systems to stop working properly.

It can seem overwhelming that so many things cause chronic inflammation and cause one another and how many ways chronic inflammation damages your body. It almost seems like there is nothing you can do. But there are many things that can be done to curb chronic inflammation and the interaction works both ways. If you improve the health of your lungs or your liver or your digestive system, your entire body benefits.

===============

PART 2 – SPECIFIC ACTIONS TO FIGHT CHRONIC INFLAMMATION

Over the next few pages many things are listed which you can do to reduce chronic inflammation. You do not need to do them all but the more things you do to reduce the inflammation the sooner you will see results and more likely you'll see a bigger change. The more you do the better. Remember also that doing something once doesn't work. These are changes that you must make for a life time.

A. The first thing you should do for improved health if you smoke or drink alcohol, is to stop. You've read what they do. They are major sources of irritation which fuels chronic inflammation and damages your body.

B. Sleep is another very important component

to good health. Besides increasing production of cortisol and decreasing production of growth hormone (which are harmful to your body) it also is associated with depression, mental fogginess and accidents. How much sleep you need probably varies but you aren't likely to find any study that suggests less than five hours per night and six hours is more common. Minimum.

C. Exercise. You don't need to run marathons or even a 10K. To reduce chronic inflammation it might be better to not run at all. Also, forget that saying, "No pain, no gain." You should never feel pain. Pant, raise your heart rate, sweat, maybe even be a little sore the next day. Those are not pain. Pain is your body saying stop.

Exercise is important because it burns sugar. It keeps the excess sugar from turning to fat cells and helps you avoid insulin resistance. It also burns off excess cortisol. Exercise also keeps all your moving parts in moving condition. Here is a saying to remember, "Use it or lose it." If you have trouble walking down the block and back, not walking isn't going to make it better.

D. Make your diet anti-inflammatory. Following are two lists to help you. The first is a list of foods to avoid. The second is a list of anti-inflammatory foods to include in your diet.

Inflammatory Foods

1. Hydrogenated oils (transfats) - Eliminate transfat from your diet. Period. This includes margarine, nondairy whipped toppings, vegetable shortening, non-dairy coffee creamer, fast food, doughnuts, crackers for starters. It's difficult to find these without hydrogenated oils. Some breads and cereals may be without transfats but not all. Regular peanut butter has transfat in it. Some natural brands have sugar. Use a natural brand without sugar. Get in the habit of checking labels for ingredients even if there is a note on the label that says "Transfat Free" because that does not mean zero. You want zero. Even some foods thought to be healthy contain transfats.

2. Corn syrup and oil - Most cola, condiments, cereals, cereal bars, yogurts, canned fruit, many sweet snacks, boxed macaroni, fruit juice, and salad dressings contain either corn oil or corn syrup. Check labels. HFCS, high fructose corn syrup, is used in a multitude of foods. It's not just blood sugar influence, but omega-6 also. It may be more difficult to

eliminate than transfat. Begin by eliminating sources with no nutritional value, like cola. If it has some nutritional value (vitamins, minerals, protein) cut use in half and avoid eating multiple things in one meal that are loaded with HFCS.

3. Sugar - Cut way back on sugary foods and eliminate added sugar - as to tea, coffee, cereal. Consider your lifestyle. If you are a pro athlete your body will burn through more sugar daily than if you are a couch potato. Include fruit juices here. They are very high in sugar and since they are already liquid they get into your blood faster.

4. Breads - Check labels for hydrogenated oil, corn oil and corn syrup. It may be difficult to find bread/bakery items without any of these but not impossible. If you don't want to eliminate completely cut the amount you eat at least in half. If you discover that you are sensitive to some component like gluten you should eliminate from your diet. Keep in mind that eating bread is eating processed food which means it becomes blood sugar fast. The less bread/baked goods you eat, the better.

5. Fast food - Most fast food is cooked in corn oil, much contains hydrogenated oil, some contains msg and high temperature cooking

like deep frying may make it more unhealthy. If you don't want to eliminate at first, cut back. Get a small instead of large, buy one instead of two and eat it less often. Make it a treat, reward or weekend special. You need to reduce fast food consumption at least in half.

6. Candy - Not necessary to eliminate, but do not eat every day and decrease portions. Find candy you like that doesn't contain corn syrup (HFCS) or hydrogenated oil.

7. Cereals - Eliminate obviously sugary cereals but read the labels, too. Some that sound healthy contain corn syrup or transfats (hydrogentated oil). Cut corn cereals way down.

8. Artificial sweeteners - Avoid in any form.

9. Processed foods - Cut back or eliminate. Essentially everything available at a supermarket is a processed food if it isn't fresh produce so this can be difficult to eliminate. When you shop look at the labels and stay away from foods with HFCS, hydrogenated oils, corn oil or artificial sweeteners. Avoid high calorie foods with no nutritional benefit. Frozen vegetables and fruits usually have greater nutrition value

than canned. When you eat noodles or other pasta or rice or potatoes, balance them by mixing with a lot of vegetables. Reduce portion sizes of processed foods. Remember part of the problem is too much sugar too fast.

10. Cooking oils - Avoid these: cottonseed, safflower, corn, soybean, sunflower, grapeseed, vegetable oils. Coconut and olive oil seem to be best for your health.

11. Alcohol - Elimination is not popular but it is best for your health. Besides the multiple problems pointed out earlier, alcohol is also high in sugar.

12. Any food you have a sensitivity to should either be eliminated or drastically reduced in your diet depending on the severity of the sensitivity. The usual suspects are peanuts, gluten, dairy, nightshade family and shell-fish but you can develop a sensitivity to anything.

If you have suspicions but aren't sure, you can do a casual test yourself. Keep a log of when you have a problem and what you ate in the hours before. Some common problems you might experience include bloating, gas, pain, sleepiness, rash, itch, diarrhea, nausea or constipation but could literally be anything. If you see a pattern of the problem occurring always after you eat a specific food take the next step. Don't eat that food for a week or more. No problem? Eat the food by itself for one meal. Have the problem? Do this a couple of times. If you have the problem when you eat the food, do one of two things – stop eating the food, or see your physician about an actual test to confirm whether you have a sensitivity.

IMPORTANT: If you have pre-diabetes or diabetes, all added sugar should be eliminated, not cut back. Sugar substitutes should be eliminated. Cut out processed foods and even natural foods with high sugar content (fruits). You need to manage your condition and fight the inflammation both and give it all you've got. Take as many steps as you can. Diabetes and pre-diabetes are serious. Don't let your disease progress!

Anti-inflammatory Foods

1. Eat more foods with omega-3, like salmon, tuna, sardines and similar cold water fish; avocado; walnuts; olive oil. In case you're wondering, olives don't have a lot of omega3 - it's in the oil - but olives are a healthy source of fiber, and vitamins and minerals.

2. Sweet potatoes are a good source of fiber, beta-carotene, manganese and vitamins B6 and C, plus complex carbohydrates which helps satisfy hunger but do not raise blood sugar levels too fast.

3. Cruciferous vegetables are broccoli, cauliflower, kale, Brussels spouts and cabbage. They are all heavy with antioxidants and other nutrients and are low in calories (sugar).

4. Spices are great inflammation fighters because they can be added to about anything. Some spices with the best anti-inflammatory action are turmeric, ginger, garlic and cilantro. Use them fresh when possible. If you have never used ginger fresh, it is found in the produce section and looks like a root (because it is). Use a potato peeler to put shavings in cooked dishes or in salads or make tea.

5. Eat berries. Blueberries, blackberries, cranberries, strawberries and raspberries are all high in antioxidants and also do other good things. For example, recent research with strawberries showed that they lower triglycerides and LDL.

6. Kelp, kombu, wakame, arame are good. These sea vegetables are anti-inflammatory,

high in anti-oxidants and provide fiber. But check the labels of seaweed snacks because some may be coated with vegetable oil.

7. Fermented foods like kimchee, sauerkraut and yogurt are important. They keep flora of your digestive system (beneficial bacteria) thriving which is extremely important for the health of your immune system. One word of caution for these and any very acidic food: they can be hard on your teeth. You can counteract that by rinsing your mouth with a little baking soda after you eat anything high in acid.

8. Spinach is low in calories plus high in anti-oxidants, high in many vitamins and minerals, fiber and has some omega-3. Cook lightly or eat raw. In soup, add it near the end of cooking other ingredients.

9. Papaya and pineapple aid digestion and are anti-inflammatory

10. The cantaloupe is low in calories, high in antioxidants and a very good source of many other vitamins and minerals

11. Lots of any fresh vegetable. Fresh fruits have a lot of nutritional value but they also

are loaded with sugar so eat smaller portions of fruit.

What about supplements? Can they make up for not eating right? No. Eating well is better for a few reasons. Eating is a requirement of life. Since you need to do it, do it right or as well as you possibly can. Plants have a lot of nutrients in them which still haven't been isolated. We don't know about them and they could be the real "medicine" in something like broccoli. Unless you are taking a fiber supplement you won't be getting fiber with supplements and you need it for good digestive system health.

This doesn't mean don't use supplements. Consider the word: supplement. They are to supplement the food you put into your body, not take the place of it. Think of the food as the gas going into your tank. Supplements are like an additive to boost the octane. Do your homework and find what supplements might help any condition you suffer from and use as directed. 'Condition' doesn't just mean a diagnosed disease, but also a common complaint or symptom. For example, if you are always tired, research to find what nutrient (the lack of) could possibly be responsible. Related to chronic inflammation, general supplements you might find useful are:

* omega-3
* probiotics, especially if you don't eat fermented food regularly
* a good general anti-oxidant like vitamin C
* vitamin D3

E. Reduce Stress. Remember that stress is the number one cause of cortisol production and cortisol encourages inflammation. Stress also causes the release of adrenaline which can increase production of the inflammatory chemical il-6 by as much as 40 times.

The best way to deal with stress is to not feel it. Change your attitude about problems. Learn to accept them as just part of life. Analyze them, deal with them, but don't fret or worry about them because it doesn't help and it can hurt your health. Here are some other ways to manage stress.

1. Meditate. It doesn't need to be complicated or mystical. Sit or lie comfortably. Close your eyes. Take a few deep breaths. Think about your breathing. Count each car passing outside. Listen for and count the ticks of the clock. Count backwards slowly from 100. Imagine a rose as vividly as possible and try to imagine the scent. Or do anything else

that helps you focus your mind on something neutral or pleasant.

2. Change the subject. You may not be able to sit and close your eyes but you can change what you are thinking about. Know ahead of time what you will switch your thought to. Perhaps the recent vacation and the most fun thing you did. Or your kids laughing. Or a hobby. Whenever thoughts come up to stress you but you aren't really dealing with it, switch to your pre-planned alternate thought.

3. Listen to the right music. In an mp3 player or on your computer, create a folder of songs for when you feel stressed. They may be gentle songs to help you relax. They may be more lively to energize you. Instrumentals are great but so are songs that include inspiring lyrics. Avoid any music with negative lyrics. Make more than one folder with music for different positive moods. Whenever you feel stressed or depressed, listen to your special music. This method can be easily combined with some of the other methods.

4. Learn something. Sometimes stress is caused by something we don't know. If your computer drives you nuts, would it help to take an introductory class on using it? If what

stresses you is an ongoing problem, analyze whether you could learn a skill to reduce or eliminate it.

5. Play a game. It can be something as short and simple as a quick game of solitaire. If you feel on edge about something, a game will force you to focus for a short time on something else. A few minutes away from the problem may be enough to change your perspective and raise your energy.

6. If you don't want to play a game, use any mental activity to force the stressful thoughts out for a time.   You could do the multiplication table 1 through 20 for the numbers 1- 6, for example. Do you know or are you learning a foreign language? Go through a series of vocabulary words - naming the objects around you.

7. Go back to nature. Do it literally if you can - at a park or in your back yard. If you can't get back to nature literally, do what you can. Buy recordings of nature sounds. Get some house plants and posters of nature scenes and candles or sprays that smell like nature - like flowers or evergreen trees. Combine these things with meditation and imagine yourself in nature. Research has shown that natural

surroundings are very conducive to relaxation.

Handy Re-cap of Things You Can Do To Fight Chronic Inflammation

1. Eliminate or seriously reduce processed foods from your diet.
2. Eliminate added sugar.
3. Eliminate use of corn by-products like corn oil and HFCS.
4. Eat foods with omega-3 and fermented foods regularly.
5. Eliminate transfat (hydrogenated oil) from your diet.
6. Use anti-inflammatory spices.
7. If you suspect you have a food sensitivity, test it, and eliminate the item from your diet.
8. Lose weight if you need to. Slow is better than no.
9. Exercise. Be active for at least 15 minutes every day.
10. Get enough sleep. A long night sleep is best but if you can't, then find a way to fit a nap into your day.
11. Reduce the stress in your life by reducing the causes or learn to counter it's effects.
12. Stop smoking.
13. Stop drinking alcohol.

Does the old saying "Anything is better than nothing" apply to fighting chronic inflammation? Maybe. If you have no specific illness it might help put off problems if you make small changes.

If you already have a problem, though, (diagnosed or undiagnosed) you need to do all that you can right now to help your body begin to work properly. There is a lot of anecdotal evidence that many (maybe all?) conditions can be reversed but you need to give it all you have, not just fool around at the edges. Dive in. Do all you can and the best time to begin was yesterday. So don't wait.

If you try to make several changes and begin to feel overwhelmed, pull back just a little. For example if you begin by trying to make seven changes, just begin three changes in behavior this week. Add three more next week and then add the last.

If you need to, pare it down to one change each week until you have made all the changes you need. Remind yourself often that every change you want to make has been made successfully by other people - lots of others - and if they can do it, so can you.

Remind yourself also that this is about your life, both quality and length.

When should you start? Right now! It is never too late. Nor is it ever too early for you to begin or for you to teach your children. Give your kids a head start on good health. Teach them the principles of an anti-inflammatory lifestyle.

What are you going to do first? Right now?

==================

Please share this life saving information with others.

You can access all the sources used to gather the information in this Cheat Sheet on the supplemental info page at http://www.cheatsheetstore.com

ABOUT THE AUTHOR

Author Norma G. Jackson attended Cornell College in Mt. Vernon, Iowa for two years and graduated cum laude from the University of Maryland. She credits her quick wit and grit to her father's warped sense of humor and Cornell College's small classroom sizes of 8 to 10 students.

Mrs. Jackson lives in Bowie, Maryland, with her husband, Leroy Jackson, Jr. She has been blessed with two brilliant and beautiful daughters, Emmanuelle and Françoise, and two amazing granddaughters, Layah and Paris.

As the former wife of a high ranking Citibank official, Ms. Jackson developed her love of writing from her years of traveling through Europe, the Sub-Sahara, Central and West Africa (Niger, Burkina Faso, Cameroun, Nigeria, Côte Ivoire, Benin). People watching became a daily game to her. Her husband's assignments couldn't keep up with her rapid imagination and her thirst for 'Why?'

Mrs. Jackson's observations of others led her to discover the strategy that helped transform her own health and subsequently give birth to her book, "Eat Like A White Chick."

Contact Mrs. Jackson for comments and inquiries at AuthorNormaJ@gmail.com.

Before

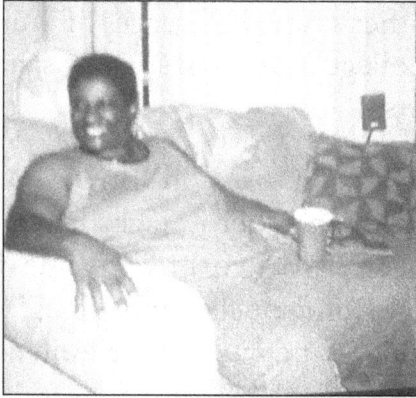

After

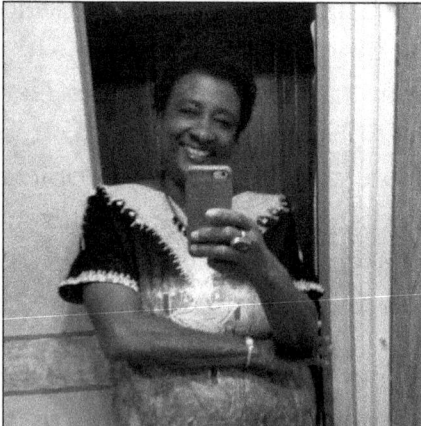